Technical Paper Series

Discussion Paper Series

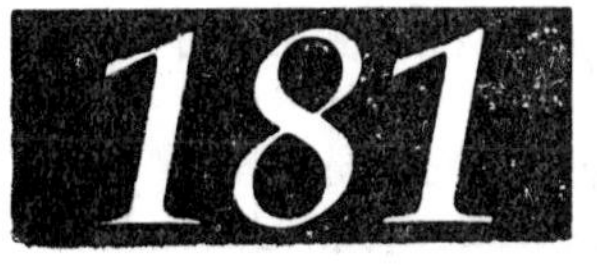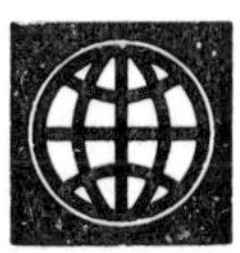

World Bank Discussion Papers
Africa Technical Department Series

Combatting AIDS and Other Sexually Transmitted Diseases in Africa

A Review of the World Bank's Agenda for Action

Jean-Louis Lamboray
A. Edward Elmendorf

The World Bank
Washington, D.C.

Discussion Papers present results of country analysis or research that is circulated to encourage discussion and comment within the development community. To present these results with the least possible delay, the typescript of this paper has not been prepared in accordance with the procedures appropriate to formal printed texts, and the World Bank accepts no responsibility for errors.

The findings, interpretations, and conclusions expressed in this paper are entirely those of the author(s) and should not be attributed in any manner to the World Bank, to its affiliated organizations, or to members of its Board of Executive Directors or the countries they represent. The World Bank does not guarantee the accuracy of the data included in this publication and accepts no responsibility whatsoever for any consequence of their use. Any maps that accompany the text have been prepared solely for the convenience of readers; the designations and presentation of material in them do not imply the expression of any opinion whatsoever on the part of the World Bank, its affiliates, or its Board or member countries concerning the legal status of any country, territory, city, or area or of the authorities thereof or concerning the delimitation of its boundaries or its national affiliation.

The material in this publication is copyrighted. Requests for permission to reproduce portions of it should be sent to the Office of the Publisher at the address shown in the copyright notice above. The World Bank encourages dissemination of its work and will normally give permission promptly and, when the reproduction is for noncommercial purposes, without asking a fee. Permission to copy portions for classroom use is granted through the Copyright Clearance Center, 27 Congress Street, Salem, Massachusetts 01970, U.S.A.

The complete backlist of publications from the World Bank is shown in the annual *Index of Publications*, which contains an alphabetical title list (with full ordering information) and indexes of subjects, authors, and countries and regions. The latest edition is available free of charge from the Distribution Unit, Office of the Publisher, Department F, The World Bank, 1818 H Street, N.W., Washington, D.C. 20433, U.S.A., or from Publications, The World Bank, 66, avenue d'Iéna, 75116 Paris, France.

ISSN: 0259-210X

In the Africa Technical Department at the World Bank, Jean-Louis Lamboray is senior public health specialist and A. Edward Elmendorf is a management specialist.

Library of Congress Cataloging-in-Publication Data

Lamboray, Jean-Louis, 1947–
    Combatting AIDS and the other sexually transmitted diseases in
  Africa : a review of the World Bank's agenda for action / Jean-Louis
  Lamboray, A. Edward Elmendorf.
       p. cm. — (World Bank discussion papers, ISSN 0259-210X ;
  181)
    ISBN 0-8213-2262-1
    1. AIDS (Disease)—Africa. 2. Sexually transmitted diseases—
  Africa. I. Elmendorf, A. Edward, 1938–   . II. International
  Bank for Reconstruction and Development. III. Title. IV. Series.
    [DNLM: 1. Acquired Immunodeficiency Syndrome—prevention &
  control—Africa. 2. Sexually Transmitted Diseases—prevention &
  control—Africa.   WD 308 L225c]
  RA644.A25L35   1992
  362.1'9697'920096—dc20
  DNLM/DLC   92-49522
  for Library of Congress   CIP

Foreword

In 1988 the Africa Region of the World Bank adopted an agenda for action on Acquired Immunodeficiency Syndrome (AIDS) in Africa. Since that time, this pandemic has become increasingly apparent and our knowledge of it has grown. It has now become critical to re-evaluate and update the Bank's original approach. The outcome of that re-evaluation is presented in this report.

The review has confirmed the scope of AIDS in Africa and its importance as a sexually transmitted disease. What was seen previously as largely a disease of urban populations is now spreading in rural areas. AIDS has become the leading cause of death among hospital patients in several African capitals. In 1992 the total number of AIDS cases in Africa is expected to reach 2.5 million.

African countries can do much to combat this disease. Information campaigns have communicated information on AIDS. New efforts need to be made to change behavior among high-risk groups. The treatment of other sexually transmitted diseases merits increasing emphasis, especially among populations with low human immunodeficiency virus (HIV) prevalence rates.

AIDS is a serious threat to Africans' health and to their countries' socioeconomic development. To combat this second threat, multisectoral programs are assuming increasing importance. The core financial and planning agencies of African governments need to focus on AIDS and its implications for development. The Bank is preparing country-specific multisectoral AIDS strategies in Africa to increase country capacity in preventing additional HIV infections and mitigating their consequences. By so doing the Bank will help African countries to combat this rising threat to development.

Ismail Serageldin
Director
Technical Department
Africa Region

Abstract

This paper reevaluates and updates the 1988 World Bank agenda for action on Acquired Immunodeficiency Syndrome (AIDS) in Africa. What was seen previously as largely a disease of urban populations is now spreading in rural areas. The paper concludes that African countries can do much to combat AIDS. New efforts need to be made to change behavior among high-risk groups. The treatment of other sexually transmitted diseases merits increasing emphasis. The core financial and planning agencies of African governments need to focus on AIDS and its implications for development.

Acronyms

AFRO	Africa Regional Office, World Health Organization (Brazzaville)
AIDS	Acquired Immunodeficiency Syndrome
AFTPN	Africa Technical Department, Population, Health and Nutrition Division
CDC	United States Centers for Disease Control
CDR	Crude Death Rate
COD	Country Operations Division
GPA	Global Programme on AIDS, World Health Organization
HIV	Human Immunodeficiency Virus
IEC	Information, Education and Communication
IMR	Infant Mortality Rate
MTP	Medium-Term Plan for AIDS Prevention and Control
NACP	National AIDS Control Program
PHRHN	Population and Human Resources Department, Population, Health and Nutrition Division
SPPF	Special Project Preparation Facility
SOD	Sector Operating Division
STD	Sexually Transmitted Disease
UNDP	United Nations Development Programme
UNFPA	United Nations Population Fund
WHO	World Health Organization

Contents

Page

Tables, Maps, and Figures

<u>**TABLES**</u>

<u>**MAPS**</u>

<u>**FIGURES**</u>

<h1 align="center">Executive Summary</h1>

The conclusion of this update of the World Bank's 1988 Technical Paper on AIDS in Africa is clear: no country in Sub-Saharan Africa can afford to delay stepping-up its response to the AIDS epidemic. The prevalence of HIV has risen — from two million cases in 1988 to more than six million in 1992 — and a whole new class of poor is taking root, consisting in part of orphans under the age of ten years old who are expected to number ten million or more by the turn of the century. The current and potential situation makes it all the more urgent for the Bank to strengthen and broaden its "Agenda for Action on AIDS and other STDs in Africa."

The worsening epidemiological situation is confirmed by reports of significant increases in the HIV infection rate in virtually all African countries and all socioeconomic levels. Nor is infection confined to urban areas. Some countries are reporting increases in the rate of infection among rural populations, and other countries are expected to suffer similar increases. The evidence concerning mortality consequences: AIDS has become the leading cause of death in adult males and the second cause among women in several capital cities, a trend evidenced throughout West Africa. The potential for spread appears high, and experts are now predicting that Sub-Saharan Africa will have a total of ten million HIV infections by 1994. Although the rate of growth of the infection is expected to eventually stabilize, the level at which this will happen depends on many factors — including sexual behavior, the level of other sexually transmitted diseases, and gender differences in high-risk behavior — all of which require immediate attention to promote stabilization.

Few would now dispute that AIDS has become a long-term problem, but its precise scope is not yet fully understood. Despite the work that has been done since 1988, information is poor concerning transmission processes and probabilities, the incubation period of the disease, variability of infectiousness, the behavior of the exposed populations, and many other aspects of the disease. Consequently, the demographic impact is difficult to predict. Although AIDS-related mortality is clearly on the rise, for example, demographic research indicates that this will have limited effect on population growth in Sub-Saharan Africa because of the continued high fertility in the region. Population structure will be only moderately affected since mortality is increasing among both adults and children, although, the number of orphans in Africa is expected to rise.

HIV infection already ranks among the top five health problems in Africa's urban populations and is exacerbating the risk of other endemic diseases, such as tuberculosis. Transmission of HIV infection also appears to be facilitated by the presence of other sexually transmitted diseases. AIDS is draining scarce resources from other curable diseases and from much-needed long-term efforts to build health systems. AIDS control is now the target of a significant proportion of government health expenditures, and manpower and facilities are being swamped with AIDS-related tasks. African countries urgently need help in coming to grips with these resource issues.

The socioeconomic issues are of no less concern. The most economically productive age group is being hard hit, in many cases leaving surviving family members without means of support. Children's schooling, health care, and other life opportunities are bound to be affected, as is the quality of life of the elderly. Since AIDS affects adults in their prime productive years across all social levels, labor shortages may be experienced in many sectors, regions, and job categories. As the epidemic spreads in rural areas, food security may also be affected.

Despite considerable progress in increasing public awareness of the disease, promoting condom use, and securing a safer blood supply, efforts need to be refocused in light of information that has surfaced in the past three-and-a-half-years. Researchers and program managers need to learn more about core groups that appear to be the main transmitters of the disease, the close tie with other STDs, and the importance of not draining all resources away from other urgent health problems. More work needs to be done to determine the economic impact of the disease and to plan support for the most severely affected segments of society. As with all major disease control programs, high priority remains on strengthening the health infrastructure and devising an optimal mix of prevention and coping programs.

Through its Global Program on AIDS, the World Health Organization (WHO), is linking the countries of Sub-Saharan Africa to meet the challenges of the epidemic, but its priorities need to be reviewed and refined. With this report, the World Bank has re-evaluated its agenda on AIDS and other STDs in Africa. This is not to say that substantial progress has not been made. The Bank has extensive studies underway on the economic impact of the disease, on the channels through which the AIDS epidemic may affect key sectors of the economy (notably agriculture and industry), and on methods of developing infrastructures to provide information and education about STD/HIV infection. Countries have been informed of the Bank's increasing attention to AIDS, to encourage these countries to add STD/HIV issues to their own policy agendas, to support seminars on related issues, and to collaborate with the World Health Organization in research and other activities related to AIDS and other STD prevention and control.

Some changes in the Bank's agenda are in order. First, additional emphasis is required to coordinate AIDS work with other programs, such as those connected with population issues and safe motherhood, and to inform staff in all sectors of the current and potential impact of STD/HIV. Second, the Bank has confined its AIDS-related lending to currently affected countries and has done little to initiate prevention in countries in which the risk of spread is high. So far, current prevention methods have overlooked the association with conventional STDs.

The Bank's strategy must now reflect its recognition that AIDS represents a serious threat to health and to economic development in Sub-Saharan Africa. Its agenda for research and fieldwork should be expanded to include policy dialogues on the impact of AIDS on development in seriously affected countries. Work on the demographic impact, for example, needs to be expanded well beyond the question of population growth and fertility to the effect on households in various sectors. The emphasis on population policies and programs must continue, of course, since adult survivors will have to bear the burden of raising the children of deceased family members, and information about safe sexual behavior should be made part of family planning services. The Bank's Country Departments should focus increasing attention on countries in which the opportunity to stem the epidemic is strong, notably those with high levels of STDs and low levels of HIV. Such interventions should be a continuing concern of population, nutrition, and health projects in Africa. In projects in which STD/HIV components are not incorporated, at an early stage in the Project Cycle the task manager should be required to justify the reasons why components for HIV and other STDs are not included. This will ensure that the AIDS issue has *not* been overlooked. Control programs need continuing financial support, which can be strengthened through further collaboration with WHO programs and other groups.

Recent experience suggests that the Bank's attention to AIDS-related problems must not overshadow the other important population, health, and nutrition issues on its agenda in Africa. Whatever resources are directed toward the vast and complex AIDS situation, their allocation must be based on clear priorities regarding the long-term development of health care systems in the region. Despite the rising levels of HIV seropositivity and AIDS cases, AIDS is being prevented today in Africa. Prevention will be reinforced by improved testing and counseling facilities and by educating uninfected adolescents — a group particularly at risk. The Bank and other donor organizations will continue to seek ways of contributing most effectively in this war of survival in Africa.

In August 1988 the Africa Technical Department issued a Technical Paper on AIDS outlining the Bank's Agenda for Action on AIDS in Sub-Saharan Africa.[1] The following paragraphs provide an update on the issues discussed in that paper, the action taken by the Bank since then, the Bank's revised strategy in the wake of that action, and the current and likely AIDS situation in Africa.

HOW SERIOUS IS THE AIDS EPIDEMIC IN AFRICA? AN EPIDEMIOLOGICAL UPDATE

Since 1988, the AIDS epidemiological situation in most of Sub-Saharan Africa has deteriorated. The August 1988 AIDS Strategy Paper, citing World Health Organization (WHO) estimates, stated that well over 2 million people in Africa were infected by HIV. In September 1990 the figure had risen to an estimated 5 million HIV-infected adults, with 70,000 officially reported and 600,000 estimated cumulative cases. WHO staff expect the cumulative total to reach upward of 2.5 million cases by 1992 and predict that about two-thirds of these cases will be among the most economically active age groups (fifteen to forty-nine years). The implications of this are two-fold: a devastating effect on the victims and a lagged but significant effect on socioeconomic development.

Infection rates among the general population and the groups at risk of contracting AIDS have increased in virtually all African countries. In 1987-88 20 to 30 percent of adults were infected with HIV in the worst-affected urban areas, notably, northwest Tanzania, Rwanda, and Uganda. Since then, the seroprevalence rate among pregnant women in Kigali, for example, has risen from 18 percent to an estimated 30 percent. Contrary to expectations in 1988, data from Tanzania, Uganda, and Côte d'Ivoire indicate that rural populations are rapidly becoming infected, and it is now generally expected that HIV will spread in many rural areas, although at a slower pace. AIDS has become the major cause of death among hospital patients in several African capital cities — Abidjan, Kinshasa, Kampala, Kigali, and Lusaka. Tables 1 and 2 show HIV-1 and HIV-2 [2] seroprevalence rates (the proportion of individuals who have antibodies to HIV) by residence and risk factor, and Maps 1 and 2 show the level of HIV infection in urban populations.

The potential for the further spread of HIV appears high. In Abidjan HIV-1 seroprevalence in low-risk groups was less than one percent in 1987

| | CAPITAL/MAJOR CITY | | OUTSIDE MAJOR CITY | |
	LOW-RISK GROUP	HIGH-RISK GROUP	LOW-RISK GROUP	HIGH-RISK GROUP
*Angola	1.3 a	14.2 a	-	-
*Benin	0.1	4.5	6.7	-
Botswana	0.8 c	1.2 c	0.1 c	-
*Burkina Faso	1.7 b	16.9 a	3.1 a	44.7 a,b
Burundi	17.5	18.5 b	-	-
*Cameroon	1.1	8.6	0.4	-
*Cape Verde	0.0	0.0	-	-
Central African Rep.	7.4	20.6	3.7	7.9
Chad	0.0	-	0.0	-
Comoros	-	0.1	-	-
Congo	3.9	34.3 b	1.0	-
*Djibouti	0.3	2.7	0.0 b	-
*Equatorial Guinea	0.3	-	0.3	-
Ethiopia	2.0	18.2	0.0	-
*Gabon	1.8	-	0.8	-
*Gambia, The	0.1	1.7 a	-	0.0 b,c
*Ghana	2.2	25.2	-	-
*Guinea	0.6 a	-	0.2	-
*Guinea-Bissau	0.1	0.0 b	0.0	-
*Ivory Coast	8.5 a	23.8 a	3.3 a	-
Kenya	7.8	59.2	1.0	-
Lesotho	0.1	-	-	-
Liberia	0.0	0.0 b	0.0 c	-
*Madagascar	0.0	0.0 b	-	-
Malawi	23.3	55.9	-	-
*Mali	0.4	23.0 a	-	-
*Mauritania	0.0 b	0.0	-	-
Mauritius	0.0	-	-	-
*Mozambique	1.1	2.6	0.8	-
*Namibia	2.5	-	-	-
Niger	-	5.8	-	-
*Nigeria	0.5	1.7	0.0	0.5
*Rwanda	30.3	79.8 b,c	1.7	-
*Sao Tome & Principe	0.0	-	-	-
*Senegal	0.1 a	2.3 a	0.0 b	-
Seychelles	-	-	-	-
*Sierra Leone	3.6 a	2.7 a	-	-
Somalia	0.0	0.4	-	-
South Africa	0.1	3.2	-	-
Sudan	0.0	16.0 b	-	-
Swaziland	0.0 b,c	-	-	-
*Tanzania	8.9	38.7	5.4	11.7
Togo	-	-	-	-
Uganda	24.3	86.0 b	12.3	76.0 b
Zaire	6.0	37.8	3.6	17.7
Zambia	24.5	54.0 b	13.0 b	13.0 b
Zimbabwe	3.2 c	-	1.4	6.6 b

- No data found.
* See Table 2 data.
a Rate represents infection with HIV-1 only and dual infection (HIV-1
   & HIV-2).
b Data are best available but are not necessarily reliable due to small
   sample size (<100).
c Data refer to prior to 1986.

Notes: High risk -- prostitutes and clients, STD patients, or other
        persons with known risk factors. Low risk -- pregnant women, blood donors,
        or other persons with known risk factors.

Source: Adapted from "Recent HIV Seroprevalence Levels by Country: February, 1991,"
Health Studies Branch, Center of International Research, U.S. Bureau of the Census,
Washington, D.C.

Table 2. ESTIMATES OF HIV-2 SEROPREVALENCE BY RESIDENCE AND RISK FACTOR, FOR AFRICAN COUNTRIES. CIRCA 1990

	CAPITAL/MAJOR CITY		OUTSIDE MAJOR CITY	
	LOW-RISK GROUP	HIGH-RISK GROUP	LOW-RISK GROUP	HIGH-RISK GROUP
*Angola	1.3 a	13.7 a	-	-
*Benin	-	3.7	0.9	-
*Burkina Faso	0.0 b	22.8 a	1.9 a	23.7 a,b
*Cameroon	0.0	0.7	0.0	-
*Cape Verde	1.4	8.2	-	-
*Djibouti	-	0.0	-	-
*Equatorial Guinea	0.0	-	0.0	-
*Gabon	0.3	-	0.0	-
*Gambia, The	1.7	25.6 a	-	3.2 b,c
*Guinea	0.2 a	-	0.0	-
*Guinea-Bissau	6.5	25.6 b	4.7	-
*Ivory Coast	3.2 a	17.2 a	2.1 a	-
*Madagascar	0.0	-	-	-
*Mali	1.4	27.4 a	-	-
*Mauritania	0.0 b	0.0	-	-
*Mozambique	2.2	1.1	-	-
*Namibia	0.0	-	-	-
*Nigeria	1.2	0.9	0.1	0.7
*Rwanda	0.0	-	0.0	-
*Sao Tome & Principe	0.0	-	-	-
*Senegal	0.1 a	10.0 a	0.0 b	-
*Sierra Leone	5.0 a	1.8 a	-	-
*Tanzania			0.1	0.3

- No data found.
* See Table 1 for HIV-1 data.
a Rate represents infection with HIV-2 only and dual infection (HIV-1 & HIV-2).
b Data are best available but are not necessarily reliable due to small sample size (<100).
c Data refer to prior to 1986.

Notes: High risk -- prostitutes and clients, STD patients, or other persons with known risk factors.   Low risk -- pregnant women, blood donors, or other persons with known risk factors.

Source: Adapted from "Recent HIV Seroprevalence Levels by Country: February, 1991," Health Studies Branch, Center for International Research, U.S. Bureau of the Census, Washington, D.C.

Tab2.wk1/dt

Map 1

African HIV-1 Seroprevalence for High-Risk Urban Populations

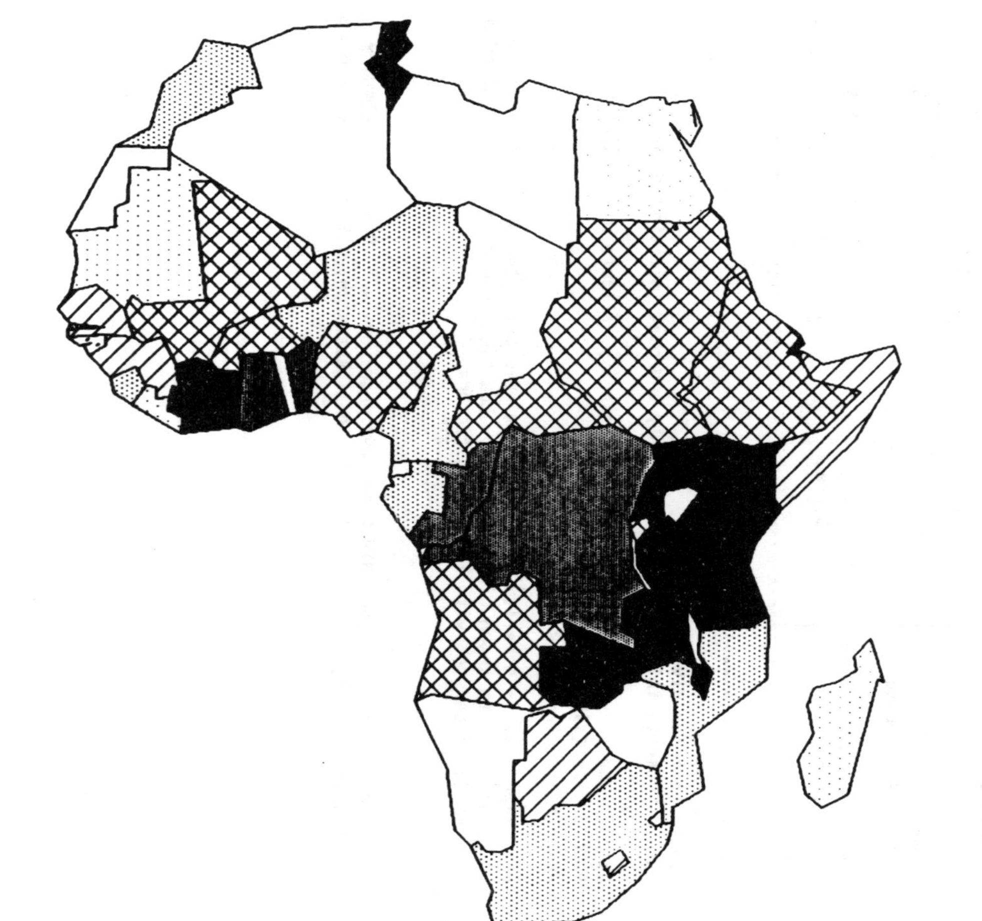

HIV/AIDS Surveillance Data Base
CIR / U.S. Bureau of the Census
April, 1992

Map 2

African HIV-1 Seroprevalence for Low-Risk Urban Populations

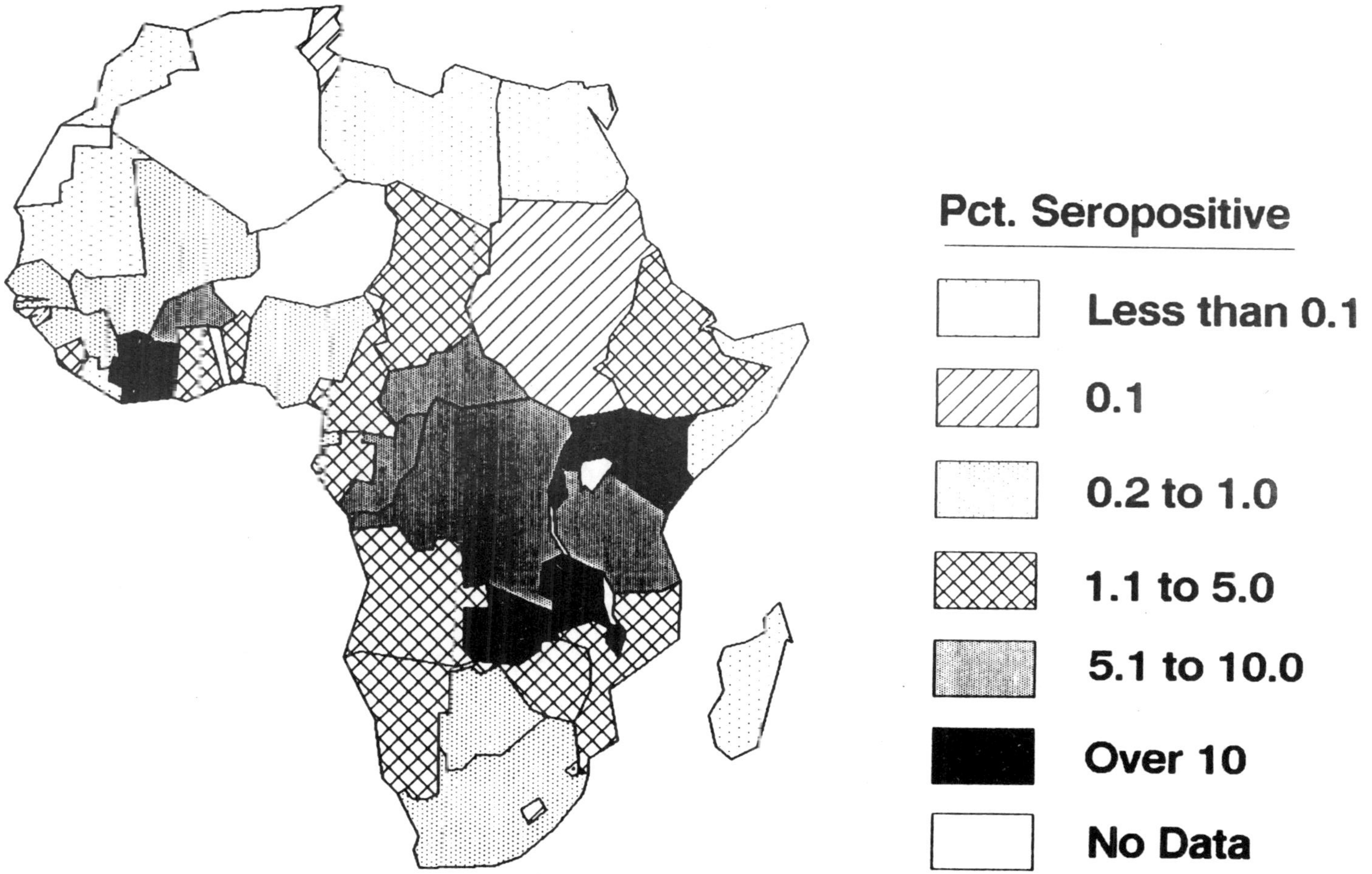

HIV/AIDS Surveillance Data Base
CIR / U.S. Bureau of the Census
April, 1992

compared to 8.5 percent in 1990.[3] Reflecting this increase, AIDS has become the leading cause of death in adult males, and the second leading cause among women. This pattern is being observed throughout West Africa, where a HIV-1 epidemic is under way in many large cities. Table 3 provides data on the current level of HIV infection and the potential for further spread in African countries. The potential for further spread is assessed along various factors, notably:

- The incidence of HIV infection in urban populations. The urban epidemic might eventually spread into rural areas through interaction between towns and villages.

- Current HIV prevalence among prostitutes and other high-risk groups. Prostitutes represent a "core group" of HIV transmitters, (see Table 4).[4] Other identifiable core groups such as clients of prostitutes, truck drivers, and the military are active in transmitting the virus to prostitutes and other partners.

- The frequency of conventional STDs, such as syphilis and gonorrhea, among the general population, pregnant women and persons seeking STD services. The frequency and distribution of STDs reflect sexual behavior patterns conducive to HIV transmission, and studies suggest that several conventional STDs facilitate HIV transmission.

According to the available data (see Table 3), twelve African countries — Cameroon, Djibouti, Ethiopia, Gabon, Gambia, Ghana, Guinea, Lesotho, Madagascar, Nigeria, Somalia, and Swaziland — have a low level of HIV infection and known high levels of STDs. The epidemic appears to have a high potential for further growth in these countries. This should become the focus of World Bank attention.

AIDS is now an urgent problem. The number of cases is rising, yet information about the epidemiology of the disease is still poor.[5] While the HIV infection is expected to eventually stabilize in each population affected, there is already limited evidence that the seroprevalence rate among pregnant women and blood donors may be leveling-off in Kinshasa at about 6 to 7 percent. The level at which it will stabilize, however, will depend on a number of variables, including sexual behavior, level of other STDs, and gender differences in high-risk behavior. By influencing these variables now, countries can influence the eventual stabilization level. But these responses must be sustainable.

Indicators of Current and Potential Spread of HIV by Country,
Based on HIV and STD Prevalence, 1990

	STD Prevalence [1]		
	HIGH	MED-LOW	UNKNOWN
Medium/High Urban HIV (> 3%)	CAR (I) KENYA (I) RWANDA (I)* ZAMBIA (I)*	ZAIRE (I) ZIMBABWE (II)	BURUNDI (I)* CONGO (I) COTE D'IVOIRE (I)* MALAWI (I)* SIERRA LEONE (III) TANZANIA (I)* UGANDA (I)*
Low Urban HIV (< 3%)	CAMEROON (II) DJIBOUTI (III) ETHIOPIA (II) GABON (II) GAMBIA (III) GHANA (II) GUINEA (III) LESOTHO (III) MADAGASCAR (III) NIGERIA (II) SOMALIA (II) SWAZILAND (II)	SENEGAL (II) SUDAN (III)	ANGOLA (III) BENIN (III) BOTSWANA (I) BURKINA FASO (I) CAPE VERDE CHAD (III) EQ. GUINEA (III) GUINEA-BISSAU (I)* LIBERIA (III) MALI (III) MAURITANIA (III) MAURITIUS MOZAMBIQUE (II) NAMIBIA SAO TOME (III) TOGO (III)
Unknown			COMOROS NIGER SEYCHELLES TOGO

Notes: Shading denotes priority; particular attention is merited to low-HIV/medium-high STD countries.

[1] As estimated from data on the prevalence of syphilis and gonorrhea in pregnant women or urban population samples.

* denotes an urban HIV seroprevalence $\geq$ 10%.

Numerals in parentheses indicate country classification in the 1988 strategy paper:

I. Countries with a high level of HIV infection;
II. Countries with a low level of HIV infection and a high rate of other STDs;
III. Countries with a low level of HIV and an unknown rate of other STDs.

Level	Country	
High (> 20%)	Burkina Faso Congo Ethiopia Guinea-Bissau Mali Senegal Uganda Zambia	CAR Cote d'Ivoire Gambia Malawi Rwanda Tanzania (West) Zaire Zimbabwe
Medium (> 5% and < 20%)	Benin Ghana Nigeria Tanzania (except West)	Cameroon Niger Sudan (South)
Low (< 5%)	Djibouti Liberia Madagascar Somalia	
Unknown	Angola Burundi Chad Equatorial Guinea Guinea Mauritania Mozambique Sao Tome Sierra Leone Swaziland	Botswana Cape Verde Comoros Gabon Lesotho Mauritius Namibia Seychelles Sudan (North) Togo

Source: US Bureau of the Census. 1992. *AIDS/HIV Surveillance Database.* Center for International Research, Washington, D.C.

CONSEQUENCES OF THE AIDS EPIDEMIC

The 1988 Strategy Paper (paragraphs nine to eighteen) stated that AIDS would seriously affect many African economies. Since then, the scope of its demographic, health, and economic effects has become clearer.

Demographic Consequences

AIDS will affect mortality, possibly fertility, the rate of population growth and the age structure. Mortality estimates can be made if we know precisely the HIV prevalence in the country. However, the future level of HIV is difficult to predict and mortality rates cannot be estimated with accuracy for the long term. Various models have been developed to estimate mortality using assumptions that have yet to be tested for their validity. Fertility rates are difficult to estimate since no one can say how people will react to AIDS in their family decisions.

Mortality. The scope and intensity of the impact of AIDS on mortality will depend on the long-term evolution of the epidemic. This will be governed by factors, such as transmission processes and probabilities, incubation period, variability of infectiousness, and the behavior of the exposed population (pairing behavior, sexual practices, other behavior affecting exposure to the virus). Although the epidemiology of AIDS may be similar in various settings, behavioral differences make it particularly difficult to arrive at a clear understanding of the disease. Behavior may change in the future, with the result that current assumptions may not hold. It is little wonder, then, that differences in seroprevalence are difficult to explain — in 1989, for example, HIV-1 seroprevalence among all pregnant women in Kinshasa was 6.0 percent in contrast to 30.3 percent in the same group in Kigali. To complicate matters even further, the long-term prevalence of HIV cannot be forecast in any society without taking into account the prevalence of other STDs such as syphilis, which can serve as a predictor of HIV seroprevalence (and facilitator of HIV infection): it may be assumed with some confidence that societies with the highest rates of conventional STDs present the greatest risk for the spread of HIV.

What *can* be predicted with reasonable accuracy is the impact of a known level of HIV prevalence on mortality at the present and in the near future. Currently, overall mortality in Africa among those *fifteen to forty-five years of age* is about five per thousand per year. Assuming a seroprevalence rate of one percent in 1987 (such is the case for Luanda, Ouagadougou, and some rural parts of Cote d'Ivoire), adult mortality is expected to increase twenty-five percent by 1992. A five percent seroprevalence rate would mean a fifty percent increase in adult mortality (as in some rural areas of Tanzania and in Kinshasa), ten percent seroprevalence would mean a 100 percent adult mortality increase (in Lusaka), and 20 percent seroprevalence would push adult mortality up 200 percent (16.4

in Blantyre, 16.3 in Bujumbura, 24.3 in Kampala; Figure 1). [6] In the age group *five and younger,* AIDS is expected to contribute ten to fifty deaths per thousand, but in some areas it will reach 100 per thousand in this age group (see Figure 2).

Fertility. The potential impact of AIDS on fertility has not been studied. Current population projection models assume that AIDS will have no impact on fertility which is expected to continue to decline gradually, as would be the case without AIDS. Yet the issue merits investigation. Crude birth rates are influenced by the proportion of women of childbearing age and the total fertility rate. The proportion of women of childbearing age is not likely to vary significantly because their high mortality rates will be partly offset by increased infant and childhood mortality. What AIDS will do to individual fertility decisions is unclear. Couples raising many children from deceased family members might want to limit their own family size. Yet, there are already anecdotal reports from severely-affected countries that couples experiencing numerous child deaths from AIDS want to have more children. Young adults might get married earlier to avoid high-risk sexual behavior, thereby increasing their fertility. Because of the long incubation period of AIDS, women infected with HIV but unaware of their status are likely to conceive several children before they develop AIDS and die. Once knowing that they are infected, some women might decide to stop conceiving to avoid transmitting the infection to newborns. Other women, especially the childless, might be more inclined to conceive. For these women, it might be worth taking the risk of giving birth to an HIV-infected child. In Africa the 30 to 50 percent probability that the child of a seropositive mother would be born HIV seropositive and die of AIDS within two years has to be compared with the current 20 percent probability that any infant will die before age five. The effect of AIDS mortality on dependency ratios also deserves attention.

Population Structure. The impact of AIDS on population structure will be minor because it will increase the mortality of both adults and children. The number of orphans will rise dramatically during the 1990s as a result of the children who are born to HIV-positive mothers but who are not infected themselves, as well as the children born before their mothers became infected. It is estimated that in high-fertility countries in Eastern Africa, for every mother dying of AIDS three children become orphans. More than ten million children under the age of ten are expected to become AIDS-bereaved orphans in Africa during the 1990s.

Rate of Population Growth. Most demographic modelers agree that the impact of HIV prevalence on population growth in Sub-Saharan countries will be moderate. Bongaarts (1988) first showed that the population growth rate would only be about one percent lower, even if a country's HIV prevalence level was

Figure 1. Projected Increase in Adult Mortality Attributable to AIDS, Sub-Saharan Africa, 1992

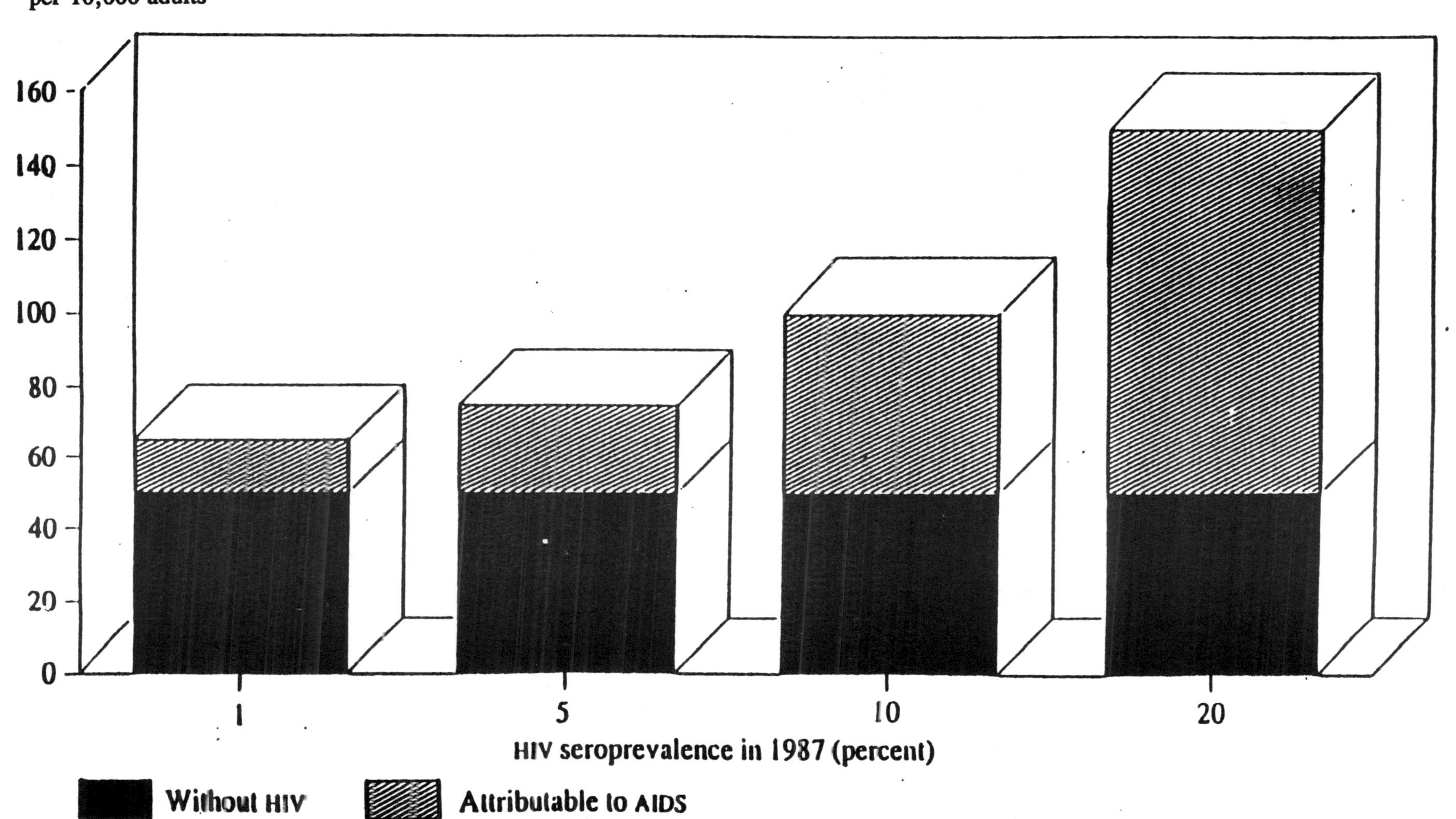

Source: Chin, J. "Epidemiology and Projected Mortality of AIDS." in Feachem, Richard G., Jamison, Dean T., eds., 1991. *Disease and Mortality in Sub-Saharan Africa.* Oxford: Oxford University Press.

Figure 2. Projected Increase in Under-Five Mortality Attributable to HIV/AIDS, Sub-Saharan Africa, 1992

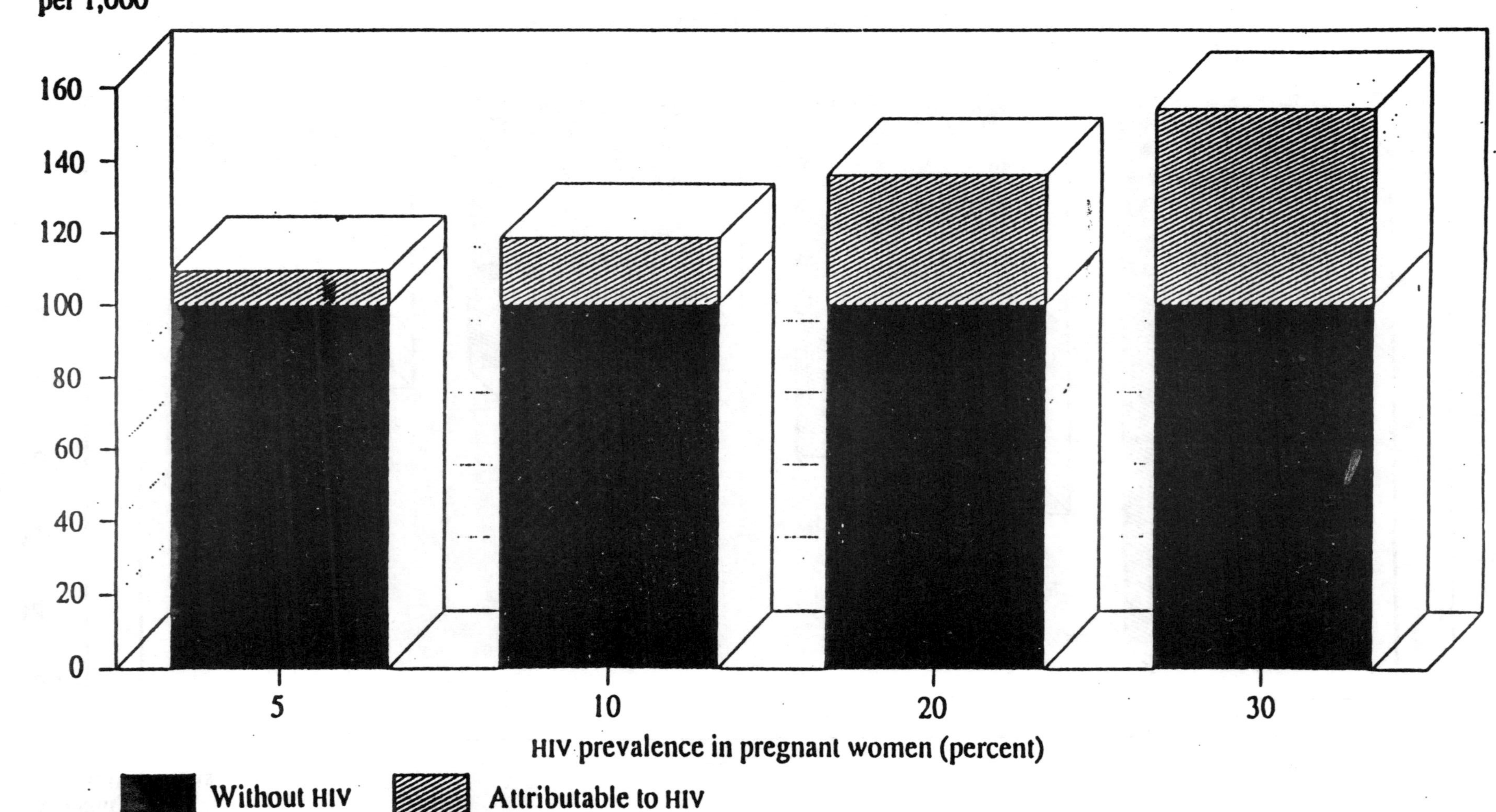

Source: Chin, J. "Epidemiology and Projected Mortality of AIDS." in Feachem, Richard G., Jamison, Dean T., eds., 1991. *Disease and Mortality in Sub-Saharan Africa.* Oxford: Oxford University Press.

to reach 20 percent — a level twice that of Uganda today (Figure 3). Because so little is known about the spread of HIV, modelers have often created "worst case" scenarios to find upper limits to the spread of the disease and its effects on population. Such scenarios usually assume no change in sexual behavior and no medical interventions, although there are indications that in some countries behavior is already changing. Among the results generated by a selection of the more well-known models applied on African countries or patterns, Anderson and others (1988) found effects high enough to generate negative population growth. Their work has been criticized for assuming transmission rates not consistent with what is known about the spread of the disease. Other models, while finding serious effects on infant mortality and life expectancy, have shown only moderate effects on population growth. This can be explained by the fact that even in the worst affected countries, most of the population will be free of the disease and unlikely to limit family size significantly.   The pattern of early and high fertility in Sub-Saharan countries means that infected women are likely to have borne several children before dying of AIDS.

Health Consequences

When estimated by the number of discounted productive healthy years of life lost per capita, HIV infection ranks among the top five health problems in urban populations with a moderate to high prevalence of HIV. The others are measles, malaria, gastroenteritis, and birth injury.[7] Even in low-endemic situations, HIV infection ranks among the twenty most important diseases by the criterion of discounted healthy years of life lost. The burden of conventional STDs in urban areas is a substantial portion of the entire disease burden on the urban population (see Figure 4).

HIV infection is having an impact on other endemic diseases. The preliminary reports about tuberculosis referred to in the 1988 Strategy Paper have been confirmed. A substantial increase in tuberculosis cases has been documented in several African countries (for example, Malawi, Tanzania, and Uganda), and the incidence of tuberculosis in people already carrying the tubercle bacillus and exposed to HIV is expected to rise because their immunity will be lower. With a growing number of sources of infection, the risk of tuberculosis in the population at large will correspondingly increase.[8]

Health Resource Allocation Issues

With the emergence of AIDS, the allocation of resources for health has been changing drastically. Some now fear that expenditures on the development of longer-term health systems and on other diseases may be reduced as a result, and that the morbidity and mortality from these diseases will grow worse. The

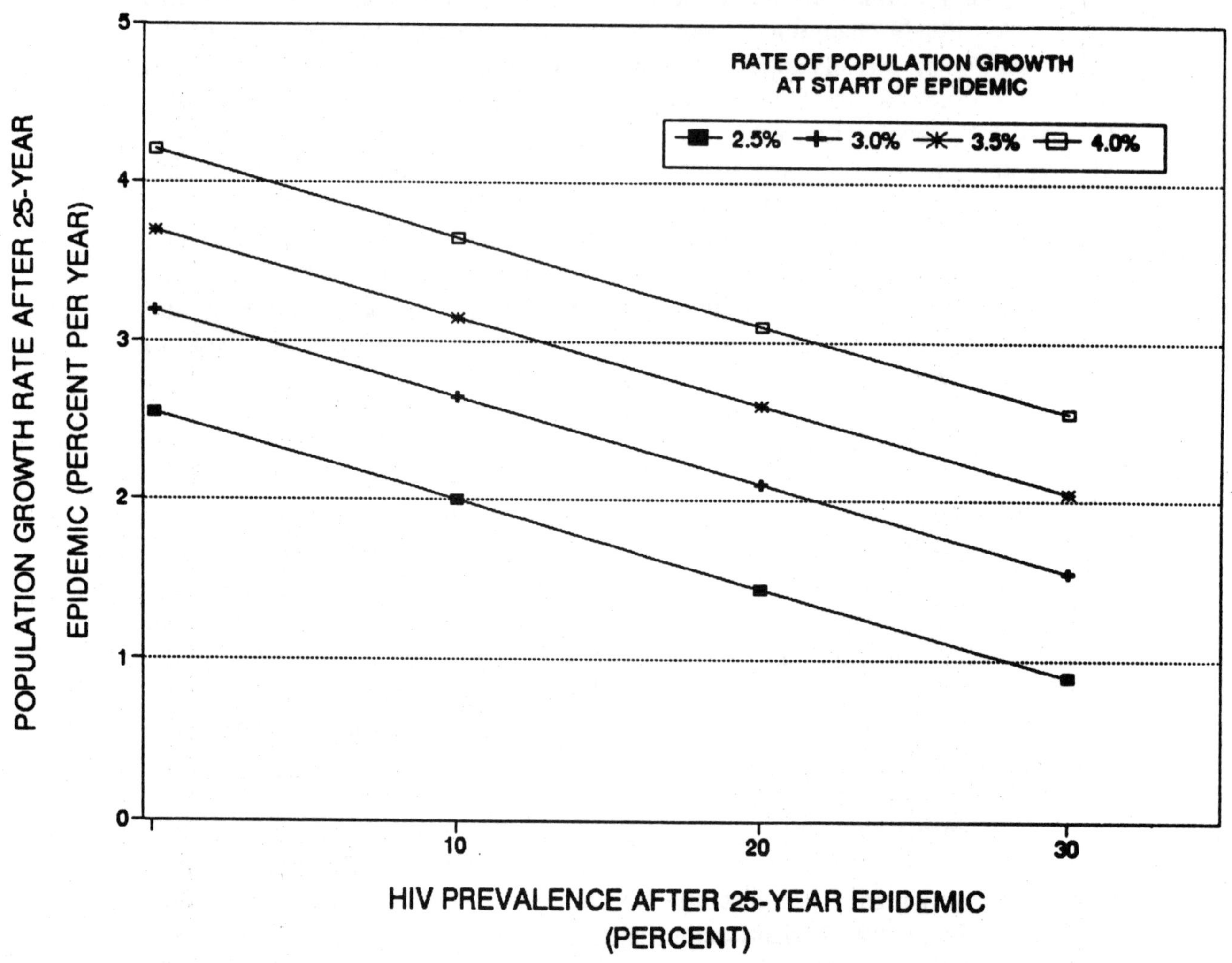

John Bongaarts. 1988. *Modeling the Spread of HIV and the Demographic Impact of AIDS in Africa.* Population Council. Center for Policy Studies. Working Papers. October 1988.

Figure 4. *STDs Share of Total Disease Burden in a High Prevalence African City*

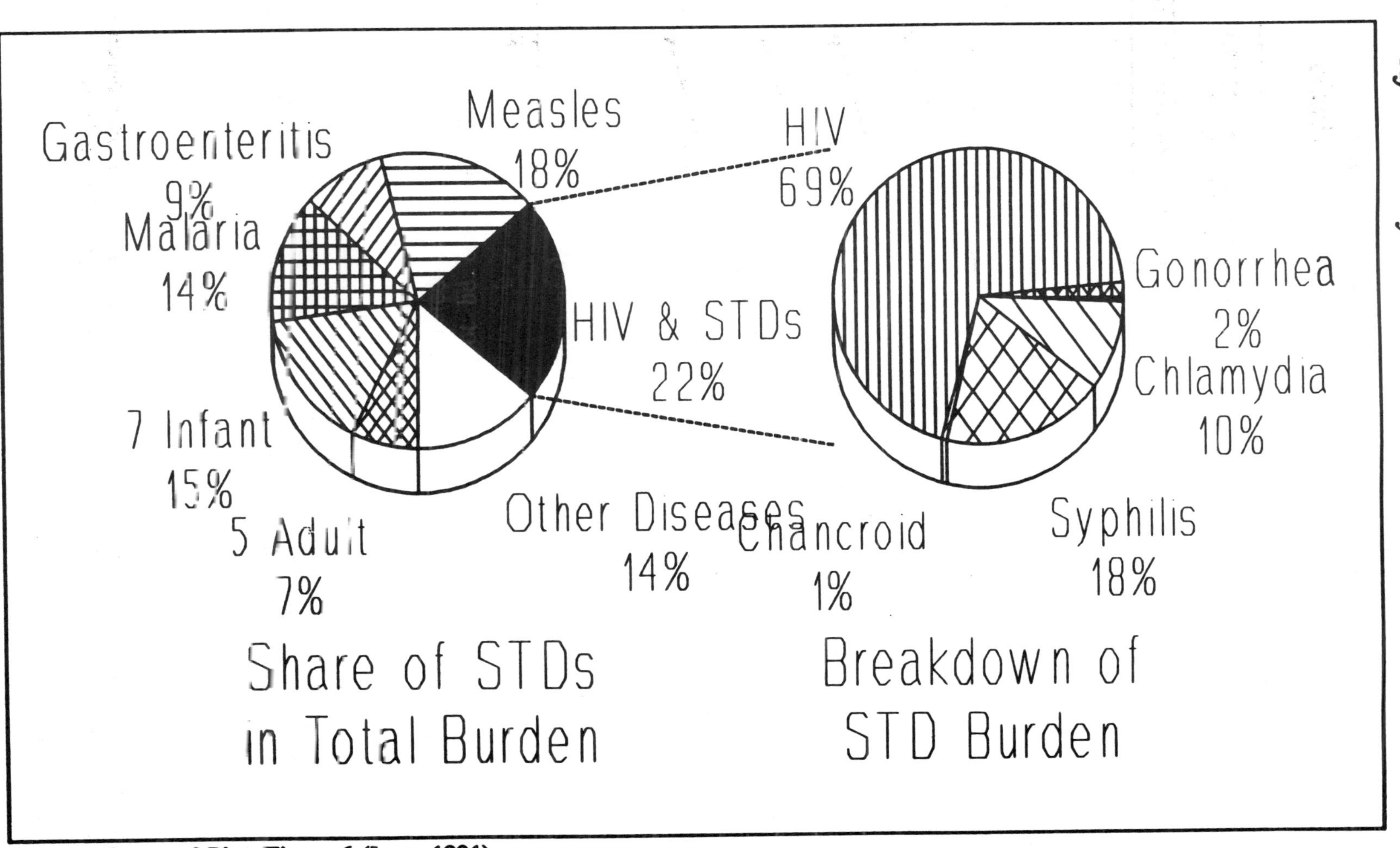

Source: Over and Piot, Figure 6 (June, 1991)

implications of these changes are particularly significant for the health systems in African countries. The medium-term plans for AIDS control prepared by African countries with WHO support, through its Global Programme on AIDS, represent a significant proportion of government health expenditures, ranging from 0.5 percent in Botswana to 21.4 percent in Rwanda, with a mean of 6 percent. Because AIDS programs supported by donors tend to offer higher salaries, scarce public health manpower is being drained from other activities and channeled into AIDS programs.

In areas with moderate to high levels of HIV seroprevalence and AIDS, hospitals are swamped with AIDS patients and are therefore becoming less effective in treating patients with curable diseases. Almost half of all hospital beds in Abidjan and the major cities in central and eastern Africa are now occupied by AIDS patients. The use of often expensive drugs for palliative relief and treatment of opportunistic infections (infections incurred when the immune system is damaged) associated with AIDS may take away resources from other hospital patients. If all AIDS patients in Tanzania were to receive care from the formal health infrastructure (assuming sufficient quantities of drugs were available), such care would consume approximately one-half of the Tanzanian recurrent public health budget for one year.[9] Estimates of the direct cost of health care per symptomatic person infected with HIV range from $132 to $1,585 in Zaire and from $104 to $631 in Tanzania (in 1987-88 U.S. dollars).[10]

We must help African countries to come to grips with the resource allocation issues raised by AIDS. Country policymakers cannot ignore the issue because the disease is fatal, nor should they concentrate resources on AIDS to the detriment of other diseases and longer-term health system development. The range of estimates of the direct cost of AIDS reflects the health care options accessible to individuals depending on their socioeconomic status and location.

Economic and Social Consequences

Since 1988, the wider implications of the AIDS epidemic have been increasingly evident at the micro and macroeconomic levels. By selectively killing people in the most economically productive age groups fifteen to forty-five years), the epidemic is creating two highly vulnerable groups of survivors — the elderly and young orphans — who have lost their principal source of support. In some areas (such as northwest Tanzania) the epidemic is stressing, to the breaking point, the traditional coping mechanisms of households and communities as they attempt to deal with catastrophic adult mortality. Surviving family members are often required to take on non-traditional activities, for which they have little or no training or experience. AIDS orphans may suffer discrimination as well as fewer life opportunities because they will not have the schooling, health care, and other amenities usually provided by parents.

The epidemic has important distributional implications. Unlike many other causes of adult death in Sub-Saharan Africa, AIDS does not spare the elite. There is evidence in several countries that infection rates among men are positively correlated with socioeconomic status. Since AIDS affects adults in their prime productive years, labor shortages may be experienced in many sectors or particular regions of the affected countries, and in some of the highly skilled job categories in urban areas. This lead to slower or perhaps negative growth in the economic sectors or regions most severely affected. Industries may have to reconsider their investment plans. As the epidemic spreads to rural areas, food security may be affected. School enrolment may suffer, as orphaned children lose the funds needed to cover these school fees and are required to contribute more time to agricultural tasks to make up for the loss of their parents' labor. In sum the AIDS epidemic means human tragedy on a wide scale in severely affected areas and a major setback for population and other development policies.

Although no major success can be reported in curbing the epidemic progress in country-level efforts is generally encouraging. For example:

- **Increased Awareness.** Survey results indicate that the knowledge and awareness of AIDS have increased substantially. Demographic and health surveys carried out in Botswana (1988) and Zimbabwe (1989) show that public education campaigns, using radio and the print media, have helped increase the public's awareness of the disease and of the role of heterosexual sex in its transmission.

- **Increased Condom Use.** The methods of social marketing adopted to promote the use of condoms (for example, in Kinshasa, Zaire) appear particularly promising. Zaire, which distributed 300,000 condoms in 1986, sold 18,000,000 condoms in 1991. However, the issue of distributing condoms in social marketing programs is far from being resolved. In Zaire one condom is sold for less than two cents, but actual costs range between two to five cents.[11]

- **Safer Blood Supply.** Progress has been made in securing safer blood supplies, particularly in the large cities. However, in some large countries (Zaire, for example) it is estimated that only 20 percent of all blood donations are tested for HIV infection. Blood screening is costly and may not be cost-effective under all circumstances.

The 1988 Strategy Paper called for action at the country level in: (a) resolving policy issues; (b) improving the efficiency of resource allocation; (c) mobilizing financial resources; (d) preparing detailed action plans; (e) strengthening country implementation capacity; and (f) improving the information base. Progress has been made in all these areas, although it has varied, by country and issue. The following specific problems now merit particular attention:

- **Coping with the Micro and Macroeconomic Impact of the AIDS Epidemic.** Irrespective of the degree of success of national programs in preventing the spread of HIV, countries with high seroprevalence will face increased adult mortality in the next ten to fifteen years because of the large number of people already infected but as yet asymptomatic. Governments urgently need to develop multisectoral policies for coping with the economic and social impact of the inevitable surge in adult morbidity and mortality. They need to analyze further the impact of the disease and current coping mechanisms, and to plan support for the most severely affected communities and sectors. Operations research is badly needed to find ways in which more care (of sound quality) can be given AIDS patients in the home and at the community level, thus by-passing the crowded hospitals. We need more information on what criteria should be used to identify the neediest of orphans (poverty level may be a better indicator of need than an AIDS-related criterion) and on what welfare programs are most effective in providing support and care.

- **Targeting Interventions to Population Groups with the Highest Payoff.** Resources for AIDS prevention and control must be allocated on at least three levels: among countries, among communities in each country, and among specific subgroups within each community. The typology of countries by level of STDs proposed in the 1988 Strategy Paper remains valid, although the classification of a few countries has changed in the light of increased knowledge.[12] Resources for prevention should be preferentially allocated to countries, communities, and target groups within communities that have low rates of HIV infection and high rates of other STDs. On these criteria, the following countries are recommended for particular attention (see Table 3).

WORLD BANK AFRICA COUNTRY DEPARTMENTS (CD)

CD1: Cameroon, Gabon, Guinea
CD2: Ethiopia, Somalia
CD3: Djibouti, Madagascar
CD4: Ghana, Nigeria
CD5: Gambia
CD6: Lesotho, Swaziland

Within communities, STD prevention and treatment programs targeted at "core transmitters" (those responsible for a disproportionately large share of HIV transmission) can have up to eight times as large a preventive impact as programs aimed at the general population. There is an urgent need to focus a larger share of AIDS and STD resources on these core transmitters in every country.

- **Establishing a Core STD/HIV Prevention and Control Program.** Each disease control program is defined by its core interventions. For instance, the Expanded Program on Immunization has its Global Immunization Schedule, and the Diarrheal Disease Control Program is built around the administration of oral rehydration. Both the WHO Global Programme on AIDS (GPA) and individual countries were initially reluctant to establish such a core program to deal with AIDS, since too little was known about the costs and effects of each intervention. In the last year it has been recognized to avoid oversized, understaffed, and unsustainable programs, priorities need to be established for interventions. Core strategies for STD/HIV prevention and control under varying conditions are proposed in Table 5.

- **Determining the Pace and Process for Coordinating HIV Activities with the Prevention and Control of Other STDs.** With the exceptions of Benin, Cameroon, Guinea, Lesotho, Senegal, Togo, Ethiopia, Tanzania and Zimbabwe, most African AIDS control programs have been developed independently of programs to control other STDs. However, a statement elaborated at a July 1990 WHO consultation on global strategies for the

Table 5: AIDS PREVENTION AND CONTROL: CORE STRATEGIES

Strategy	Condition	Objective/Goal	Target Group	Intervention	Infrastructure
A	High STD prevalence with low or high HIV	Reduce STDs as vehicle to reduce sexual transmission of HIV	Prostitutes and clients	IEC and Counseling	Community-based condom promotion and distribution
				Increase condom use	Small village pharmacies
				Detect and treat STDs	Basic health services
B	High HIV prevalence	Reduce blood transmission	Patients needing transfusion	Reduce contaminated blood	Hospital laboratories
C	High AIDS prevalence	Mitigate impact of AIDS on patients and families	Patients with AIDS	Manage opportunistic disease and symptoms at home	Outreach from basic health services
			Orphans without family support		Social support services

Note: The above strategies are *not* mutually exclusive.

coordination of AIDS and STD control programs recommended "the close coordination or, where appropriate, the combining of AIDS and STD control programs". In our view AIDS and STD programs should normally be carried out jointly. HIV infection is fundamentally an STD. Syphilis has similar transmission modes and had the same lethal outcome until the discovery of penicillin. The same prevention and control interventions apply to HIV infection and other STDs. Because STD control is a priority in its own right, HIV infection prevention and control activities should generally be incorporated into STD prevention and control. It would be unwise to concentrate only on those STDs that facilitate HIV transmission, since other STDs have a great impact on fertility and health. All people infected with STDs should be told that their sexual behavior puts them at high risk.

- **Strengthening Key Elements of the Health Infrastructure to Implement STD/HIV Prevention and Control Programs More Effectively.** High priority should be given to strengthening elements of the health infrastructure critical to the prevention and control of STD/HIV (see Table 5). In view of the urgency of controlling HIV infection and the time it takes to strengthen the infrastructure, there may be justification for continuing with vertical programs until heath systems are developed to provide a range of services effectively. The medium-term goal should, remain to integrate AIDS and other STD services into ongoing basic programs of disease prevention and health care, and to provide support to the most seriously affected segments of the population (especially orphans). Each country will need to determine the optimal mix between integrated and vertical approaches, and review it over time.

WHO'S GLOBAL PROGRAM ON AIDS (GPA)

With GPA support, as of January 1991, forty-one of the forty-three countries in Sub-Saharan Africa had set up a National AIDS Control Program (NACP) and have mobilized resources to implement the Medium-Term Plan (see Table 6). Fifteen programs were reviewed about one year after implementation was initiated and the results led WHO to revamp the program in seventeen countries. To build national AIDS programs in these countries in a matter of only three and a half years represents a high achievement.

Dr. Michael Merson, the GPA Director, described the following priorities during the Fifth Conference on AIDS in Africa (Oct. 11-12, 1990):

- Strengthen national AIDS control programs, focusing more on key interventions likely to have the greatest impact on reducing HIV transmission (condom promotion and STD treatment are obvious examples).

- Place higher priority on effective and efficient program management.

- Strengthen the social response to HIV and AIDS by recognizing that community-based organizations are key to providing this response.

- Plan now for the social and economic consequences of HIV/AIDS.

- Continue strong working relationships with United Nations Development Program (UNDP), the World Bank, UNICEF, UNFPA, UNESCO, and the European Economic Communities (EEC) and expect that over the next few years, national AIDS control programs in many African countries will be implemented as multisectoral programs.

- Build upon what has been learned about women and AIDS.

- Undertake more intervention-related studies to strengthen the technical basis of AIDS control strategies.

- Accelerate and focus research and development activities, especially with regard to new vaccines and drugs.

Since the October conference, WHO has taken action internally to increase attention to STDs and gradually merge its AIDS and STD work.

Table 6: GLOBAL PROGRAM ON AIDS: STATUS OF WHO-SPONSORED MEDIUM-TERM PLANS (MTP)
          FOR AIDS PREVENTION AND CONTROL IN AFRICA

Country or Area	Medium-Term Plan (MTP) Formulation	Mobilization of Interested Parties-Phase 1	Initial Review of Implementation	Program Formulation Phase 2	Mobilization of Interested Parties, Phase 2
Angola	Mar-89				
Benin	Aug-88	29-Jun-89	Nov-90	Nov-90	
Botswana	Jul-87	27-Jul-89	Oct-90	Feb-91	(May-91)
Burkina Faso	Mar-89	11-Oct-89	(1991)		
Burundi	Mar-88	14-Jul-88	Mar-90	Apr-90	26-Sept-90
Cameroon	Feb-88	05-Jul-88	Nov-89	Feb-90	22-May-90
Cape Verde	Apr-89	12-Jul-90			
Cent. African Rep.	Jul-88	19-Jul-88	Apr-90	May-90	
Chad	May-89	06-Nov-89	Nov-90		
Comoros	Nov-88	26-Jun-90	Mar-91	Mar-91	(May-91)
Congo	Feb-88	28-Jun-88	Nov-90	Dec-89	13-Apr-90
Côte d'Ivoire	Oct-88	20-Jun-89	Nov-90	Nov-90	
Equatorial Guinea	Jul-89	27-Feb-90	Feb-91	Feb-91	
Ethiopia	May-87	04-Aug-87	May-89	Jul-89	06-Oct-89
Gabon	Mar-89	27-Nov-89	Nov-90	Nov-90	
Gambia	Oct-88	28-Aug-89	Mar-91		
Ghana	Jul-88	04-Sep-89	Mar-91		
Guinea	Aug-89	15-Nov-90			
Guinea-Bissau	Jul-88	13-Jun-89	Feb-91	Apr-89	
Kenya	Apr-87	31-Jul-87	Jul-89	Mar-91	09-Nov-89
Lesotho	Jan-88	18-Apr-88	Feb-91	Mar-91	(May-91)
Liberia	Sep-88	31-Aug-89	(1991)		
Madagascar	Dec-89	Nov-90	(Oct-91)		
Malawi	Feb-88	29-Jun-89	Mar-90	Apr-90	02-Oct-90
Mali	Dec-88	23-Nov-89	(May-91)		
Mauritania	Feb-90	(Jan-91)			
Mauritius	Feb-89	08-Aug-89	Oct-90	Nov-90	(Apr-91)
Mozambique	Aug-87	19-Apr-88	Dec-89	Mar-90	4-Jul-90
Namibia	(Feb-91)				
Niger	Nov-88	17-Jan-90	Apr-89		
Nigeria	Feb-89	21-Mar-90	(1991)		
Rwanda	May-87	28-Jul-87	Mar-89	Jun-89	05-Mar-90
Soa Tome & Principe	Mar-90	(Mar 91)	(Dec-91)		
Senegal	Jul-87	15-Feb-88	Oct-89	Nov-89	13-Jun-90
Seychelles	Dec-88	11-Aug-88	(Jun-91)	(Jun-91)	(Aug-91)
Sierra Leone	Sep-88	(Mar-91)			
Swaziland	Oct-88	17-Apr-89	Feb-91	Mar-91	(May-91)
Tanzania	Jun-87	24-Jul-87	May-89	Jul-89	15-Nov-89
Togo	Apr-89	30-Jan-90	(Apr-91)		
Uganda	Feb-87	22-May-87	Dec-88	Jan-89	17-Jul-89
Zaire	Sep-87	11-Feb-88	Feb-90		
Zambia	Aug-87	16-Mar-88	Oct-89	Apr-90	26-Jul-90
Zimbabwe	Aug-88	25-Jul-88	Mar-90	Apr-90	15-Aug-90

* Dates given in parentheses are planned dates.

Source: World Health Organization, Global Program on AIDS, National Program Support,
         Status of Collaboration with Countries and Areas as of January 1991.

The Bank should continue its cooperation and contact with GPA, especially on analytical work. Cooperation and consultation should be sought on operational work and technical assistance.

THE BANK'S CONTRIBUTION TO STD/HIV PREVENTION AND CONTROL IN AFRICA

Country-Level and Regional Activities

Economic and Sectoral Studies. The Bank's 1988 AIDS Strategy Paper called for systematic reviews of the current and potential extent of both AIDS and STDs as part of regular sectoral work, project preparation and supervision. To help carry out these reviews, the Bank's Africa Technical Department, Population, Health and Nutrition Division (AFTPN), circulated to the Sector Operating Divisions (SODs) guidelines developed jointly with the EEC AIDS Task Force.

Although progress has been slow, several important studies are under way. Sectoral studies are addressing the AIDS issue in Tanzania and Uganda. The Tanzania study is analyzing the economic impact of the disease. The analyses are focusing on the discounted healthy years of life lost and on the development of a new model using recent output and employment data in an attempt to estimate the impact of AIDS on the labor force, GNP, savings increment, and exports. Fiscal implications will be examined nationally and in selected sectors. The study will review the alternatives for cost-effective interventions and the decentralized process for selecting these interventions according to the epidemiologic and institutional situation of districts in Tanzania. The study on Uganda will describe the channels through which the AIDS epidemic may affect key sectors of the economy and, where possible, will quantify these effects. In addition to exploring the consequences of AIDS for agriculture and industry, the study will quantify drug costs associated with AIDS, highlighting the opportunity costs of treating AIDS patients.

The AIDS study program called for in the Strategy Paper is being carried out largely as initially proposed: (a) AFTPN is collaborating with WHO/GPA on AIDS program costs and on the conceptual framework needed to integrate patient management into health care systems; and (b) Senegal and Uganda, with SPPF support, are working on a low-cost methodology of assessing STD prevalence. The initial study report, completed by WHO with the assistance of the U.S. Centers for Disease Control (CDC) is now being reviewed. WHO plans other tests worldwide.

Research. AFTPN and the Population, Health and Nutrition Division (PHRHN) of the Population and Human Resources Department have launched a three-year cooperative study of the economic impact of disease-related adult mortality on households and communities; the study is being carried out in Tanzania with the participation of Tanzanian researchers. In addition to quantifying the impact of AIDS mortality, the study will define criteria for identifying the most severely affected survivors and will estimate the costs and effects of alternative governmental and nongovernmental policies to assist them. The study's policy workshops will guide evolving national policies on survivor assistance, and the final report will estimate the macroeconomic implications of the microeconomic findings. Additional research in PHRHN, also supported by AFTPN, is using macroeconomic models to estimate directly the impact of typical epidemic scenarios on both the aggregate and sectoral growth of African economies.

Policy Dialogue. The 1988 Strategy Paper urged the Bank to convey its willingness to assist countries with high HIV prevalence to prevent and control AIDS and to help the less-affected countries by focusing on the prevention and control of STDs as a way of stemming the spread of HIV. These messages have been communicated to governments through Bank participation in MTP resource mobilization meetings, and through SOD staff. As yet, however, the Bank's efforts to put the AIDS issue on the policy agenda of low-HIV/high-STD countries have been minimal.

Lending. The Strategy Paper called for twenty-one AIDS components/projects in the Bank's operations program (fiscal 1989-92). Twenty Bank projects planned or approved for Africa in fiscal 1982-93 have AIDS components (See Table 7). These components would strengthen the management of health services, disease surveillance, and blood safety. One approved project, in Zaire, is a free-standing AIDS project. The Uganda government has requested IDA support for a multisectoral strategy and project to fight AIDS. An identification mission took place in early 1991 with full collaboration from WHO/GPA, UNDP, and other donors active in Uganda.

Donor Coordination. As of January, 1991, WHO-sponsored resource mobilization meetings had taken place for thirty-five of the forty-two African countries that have MTPs. The Bank has been represented at most of the meetings, where it has commented on the MTPs and indicated its willingness to finance AIDS prevention and control. However, African governments have been reluctant to borrow funds for AIDS programs, even on IDA terms. With the significant exception of Nigeria — a low-prevalence country — most African countries have been able to mobilize sufficient resources for their MTPs from donor grants. Some opportunities to raise the AIDS issue, such as the Niamey Safe Motherhood Conference, have been not been fully exploited.

Table 7: CONTENT OF AIDS COMPONENTS IN PLANNED AND APPROVED BANK/IDA ASSISTED PROJECTS IN AFRICA, FY 82-93

Country	Title	FY	IBRD $M	IDA $M	Strengthening Mangement	IEC	Safe Blood	AIDS Surveillance	AIDS Control	Case Management	Training	Operations Research	Integration of AIDS & STD Control
Botswana	Family Health	84											
Burundi	Health/Pop I	88		14.0		X	X	X	X		X		
Burundi	Health/Pop II	93		65.3									
Benin	Hlth Svce. Dev.	89		18.6	X				X		X		
Cameroon	Social Dim. Adj.	90	20.0										X
CAR	Health Sector	92											
CAR	Educ. IV	93											
Guinea	Pop/Health	88		19.7		X	X						
Guinea-Bissau	PHN	87		4.2			X		X	X		X	
Kenya	Population II	82											
Lesotho	Health/Pop II	90		12.1				X	X	X		X	
Malawi	PHN Sector Cr.	91		30.0									
Niger	Health	86		27.0			X						
Nigeria	IMO Health/Pop	89	27.6			X	X	X					
Rwanda	PHN II	92		26.7									
Togo	Pop/Health Adj.	91		12.0	X	X			X				
Uganda	Health Reconstr.	88		52.5		X	X			X	X		
Zaire	AIDS	89		8.1	X	X		X				X	X
Zimbabwe	Family Health	87	10.0			X							X
Zimbabwe	Family Health II	91	25.0			X							X

AFTPN, April 11, 1991, TABLE7.WK1

Relations with WHO

The Bank has consulted and collaborated extensively with GPA[13] in operational work in several African countries, attended meetings on resource mobilization for AIDS in African countries, and is providing support for studies by GPA. With Bank support, GPA has completed draft costing guidelines for AIDS programs; further efforts are needed to make this potentially valuable tool a practical reality in day-to-day STD/HIV planning activities in Africa. The Bank's Special Grants Program provided the GPA with $1 million in fiscal 1989 for the development of operational research related to AIDS prevention and control. The implementation of this research program is overseen jointly by GPA and WHO's Tropical Disease Research and Human Reproduction Programs. Although expenditures for the research areas are only just beginning, the proposals funded are important initial steps in understanding the links between the prevention and control of HIV/AIDS, tropical diseases, and reproductive health measures. The Bank authorized another grant of $1 million to GPA in fiscal 1990 under similar arrangements. Future contributions will be allocated to operations research for evaluating and refining the core strategy. WHO is gradually decentralizing operational responsibility for its AIDS work in Africa to its Regional Office in Africa, WHO/AFRO; Bank contacts on AIDS with AFRO may well need to increase.

FUTURE BANK STD/HIV WORK IN AFRICA: CONCLUSIONS AND RECOMMENDATIONS

In view of the 1988 decision to deal with AIDS using existing resource levels and the small PHN staff that has had to handle a steadily increasing work program, we conclude that the agenda in the 1988 Strategy Paper has been reasonably well implemented. However, the following shortcomings should be noted:

- In general AIDS has been incorrectly defined as an isolated issue in the health sector. AIDS work has not been sufficiently coordinated with other Programs of Special Emphasis, such as population and safe motherhood. Nor have enough resources been applied to analyzing the impact of AIDS on population and other sectors. Staff in other sectors with countrywide responsibilities have not been sufficiently informed about the current and potential impact of AIDS.

- AIDS-related lending has been confined to currently affected countries, and little has been done by the Bank to prevent AIDS in less affected countries with a high potential for spread. Prevention and control efforts have focused too much on AIDS, with the result that conventional STDs have often been neglected.

Since AIDS represents a serious threat to health, and to development in Sub-Saharan Africa, the Bank's analytical and operational agenda on AIDS should be strengthened and broadened in the following ways:

- The policy dialogue in Country Departments and with borrowers should examine the impact of AIDS on development in the seriously affected countries as well as those with a low level of HIV but high levels of STDs; this covers a total of twenty-five countries (see Table 3). An AIDS/STD Overview should be prepared before substantial dialogue is initiated. Because AIDS is affecting increasing numbers across all sectors of society, neither the analytical work nor the operational follow-up (which is both significant and multisectoral) can be handled effectively by the human resources divisions alone.

- Since AIDS affects population variables it should be included in our dialogue on population issues. Even in those countries that are most affected, the macroeconomic argument for controlling population growth remains valid. The emphasis on population policies and programs must continue, particularly since adult

survivors will have to bear the increased burden of foster children
and will have an increased incentive to limit the number of their
own children. As most adults will stay free of HIV infection, they
will continue to need family planning services.   This should
include information and advice about safe sexual behavior as part
of family planning counseling, and the distribution of condoms,
even to those clients who are more interested in preventing
STD/HIV transmission during casual sex than in preventing
pregnancies with their regular partners. In less affected countries,
we should take the opportunity during our dialogue on population
issues to highlight the effects of AIDS on development and the
benefits of preventing the epidemic at early stages.

- The Bank's Africa Country Departments should focus increasing
  attention on countries with high levels of STDs and low levels of
  HIV, because these countries represent opportunities to stem the
  epidemic.

- AIDS control should be made a part of our population program
  efforts, and the Safe Motherhood Initiative. Population projections
  produced by PHRHN need to take AIDS into account.

- The analytical agenda devoted to assessing the impact of AIDS
  needs to be strengthened and broadened. More work needs to be
  done on the demographic impact of AIDS well beyond the question
  of population growth, to determine how AIDS is affecting fertility,
  dependency ratios, and other factors. The impact of AIDS on
  households and on various economic sectors needs to be assessed
  within a macroeconomic framework. The sector work in Uganda
  should be used to develop such a framework. AIDS issues should
  appear or at least be considered in Bank-supported household
  surveys such as the SDA surveys and the DHS series financed by
  USAID.

- AIDS studies should eventually be expanded beyond PHN. Once
  our understanding of the microeconomic impact of AIDS is more
  advanced (as a result of the joint PHRHN/AFTPN study in
  Tanzania) plans for STD/HIV overviews as part of non-PHN
  sectoral studies can be initiated.

- Analytical work on methods of improving STD/HIV interventions
  should continue. The AFTPN regional study program addresses
  key issues and should continue. Sector work should include

systematic reviews of AIDS and other STDs. These reviews should be made part of the identification and appraisal of PHN projects and should feed into policy dialogue at the macro and sectoral levels. In countries singled out for priority attention, any reasons for not incorporating STD/HIV components in projects should be spelled out early in the Project Cycle.

- PHN lending should continue to focus on health policies and on the development of health systems. High priority should be given to developing those elements critical to STD/HIV control and prevention (see Table 5). Where STD/HIV control programs need support, the Bank should generally concentrate on supporting STD prevention and control. Since the health systems alone cannot cope with the AIDS/HIV epidemic, nongovernmental and community groups will need to be increasingly involved, and their roles will need to be strengthened.

- Information on AIDS should continue to be distributed to PHR staff. AIDS updates should now go to staff in Country Operations Divisions (CODs) and non-PHR SODs, as well as to those already receiving them; these updates should be made a quarterly publication.[14] AFTPN should continue to collaborate with PHRHN in organizing AIDS Working Group seminars. The composition of the Working Group should be expanded to include other SOD and COD staff.

- The Bank should continue to collaborate with GPA and the other WHO programs and groups concerned with STD/HIV control. Cooperation with WHO on AIDS in Africa should concentrate on analytical work; but consultation on operations and technical assistance should also be encouraged. The Bank should cooperate in studies and technical assistance on AIDS being sponsored by UNDP.[15]

- AIDS should not be allowed to dominate the Bank's agenda on population, health, and nutrition issues in Africa. Population and family planning programs need continued and increased attention, and health policies and systems require further work to ensure they will adjust and adapt to the full range of demographic, economic, and health realities African countries are facing in the 1990s. Maintaining the right balance will be a major challenge in allocating resources to health in Africa in the years ahead.

1. To avoid confusion with the Bank's Agenda for Action on Implementation of Population Programs in Sub-Saharan Africa, the AIDS Agenda paper is referred to in this report as the 1988 AIDS Strategy Paper.

2. There are at least two HIV strains in Africa. HIV 1, the predominant strain, is most prevalent in Central Africa, and HIV 2 is more prevalent in West Africa. HIV 2 does cause AIDS, but its incubation period (between the onset of HIV 2 infection and AIDS) is longer.

3. Data taken from HIV/AIDS Surveillance Data base compiled by U.S. Bureau of the Census for International Research.

4. "Core transmitters" is an epidemiological concept designating a relatively small group of individuals who are directly or indirectly the source of a disproportionately high number of infections. With AIDS, this is usually a result of sexual behavior. According to a recent modelling exercise, when a case of HIV infection is prevented in the core group, the total health impact is three to six times greater than preventing a case in the non-core group. See Mead Over and Peter Piot. 1991. "HIV Infection and Sexually Transmitted Diseases." June, 1991 — in Dean T. Jamison and W. Henry Mosely, eds. forthcoming. *Disease Control Priorities in Developing Countries*. New York: Oxford University Press for the World Bank, p. 37.

5. There is uncertainty among researchers about heterosexual transmission probabilities. Underlying probabilities may be quite heterogeneous. From studies on U.S. populations, the probability of transmission appears to fall in the range of .001 to .01 per contact for male to female and one-fourth to one-tenth of that from female to male contact. The presence of ulcerations appears significantly to increase transmission probabilities; they multiply the risk to males more than to females, thus roughly equalizing transmission probabilities. Some modelers have moved from using multiplier factors for STDs of 5 or 6 to between 10 and 200 for increasing the transmission probability. (Source: Memorandum of R. Bulatao, January 15, 1991.)

6. Figures obtained from WHO/GPA Surveillance, Forecasting and Impact Assessment Unit, 1990.

7. Mead Over and Peter Piot. 1991. "HIV Infection and Sexually Transmitted Diseases." June, 1991 — in Dean T. Jamison and W. Henry Mosely, eds. forthcoming. *Disease Control Priorities in Developing Countries*. New York: Oxford University Press for the World Bank.

8. Murray, C., A. Rouillon, and K. Styblo. 1990. "Tuberculosis." in Dean T. Jamison and W. Henry Mosely, eds. forthcoming. *Evolving Health Sector Priorities in Developing Countries*. World Bank, Washington, D.C.

9. See World Bank, forthcoming. *Tanzania AIDS Planning Assessment*. Washington, D.C.

10. These cost figures are from Over, M., S. Bertozzi, J. Chin, B. N'Galy, and K. Nyamuryekung'e. "The Direct and Indirect Cost of HIV Infection in Developing Countries," in A. Fleming and others, eds. 1988. *The Global Impact of AIDS*. New York: Alan R. Liss.

11. Social marketing refers to the use of commercially developed techniques to promote and market products and services subsidized for social reasons; often the social marketing organization is a nonprofit

body acting on contract with the government. The Zaire social marketing program was developed by Population Services International (1988).

12. The Strategy Paper classified countries into three groups: Group I consists of countries with a high level of HIV infection (CAR, Congo, Kenya, Uganda, Malawi, Burundi, Rwanda, Zaire, Tanzania, Zambia, Guinea Bissau, Burkina Faso, Côte d'Ivoire, and Botswana); Group II comprises countries with a low level of HIV infection and a high rate of other STDs (Cameroon, Gabon, Ethiopia, Ghana, Senegal, Swaziland, Zimbabwe, Somalia, Nigeria, and Mozambique); and Group III consists of those with a low level of HIV and an unknown rate of other STDs (Benin, Equatorial Guinea, Guinea, Togo, Mauritania, Sudan, Comoros, Djibouti, Madagascar, Liberia, Sao Tome, Sierra Leone, Chad, Gambia, Mali, Niger, Lesotho, and Angola).

13. Contacts have also been established with UNFPA on their work on AIDS.

14. This task has been assigned to a CDC staff member who to has joined AFTPN on a two-year secondment financed by the CDC.

15. UNDP has funded local studies to better understand the social circumstances of the AIDS epidemic and is initiating a global technical assistance project in Africa on how countries can address the social and economic impact of AIDS; Bank staff are consulting with UNDP on these activities.

Distributors of World Bank Publications

ARGENTINA
Carlos Hirsch, SRL
Galeria Guemes
Florida 165, 4th Floor-Ofc. 453/465
1333 Buenos Aires

**AUSTRALIA, PAPUA NEW GUINEA,
FIJI, SOLOMON ISLANDS,
VANUATU, AND WESTERN SAMOA**
D.A. Books & Journals
648 Whitehorse Road
Mitcham 3132
Victoria

AUSTRIA
Gerold and Co.
Graben 31
A-1011 Wien

BANGLADESH
Micro Industries Development
    Assistance Society (MIDAS)
House 5, Road 16
Dhanmondi R/Area
Dhaka 1209

   Branch offices:
   156, Nur Ahmed Sarak
   Chittagong 4000

   76, K.D.A. Avenue
   Kulna 9100

BELGIUM
Jean De Lannoy
Av. du Roi 202
1060 Brussels

CANADA
Le Diffuseur
C.P. 85, 1501B rue Ampère
Boucherville, Québec
J4B 5E6

CHINA
China Financial & Economic
    Publishing House
8, Da Fo Si Dong Jie
Beijing

COLOMBIA
Infoenlace Ltda.
Apartado Aereo 34270
Bogota D.E.

COTE D'IVOIRE
Centre d'Edition et de Diffusion
    Africaines (CEDA)
04 B.P. 541
Abidjan 04 Plateau

CYPRUS
Cyprus College Bookstore
6, Diogenes Street, Engomi
P.O. Box 2006
Nicosia

DENMARK
SamfundsLitteratur
Rosenoerns Allé 11
DK-1970 Frederiksberg C

DOMINICAN REPUBLIC
Editora Taller, C. por A.
Restauración e Isabel la Católica 309
Apartado de Correos 2190 Z-1
Santo Domingo

EGYPT, ARAB REPUBLIC OF
Al Ahram
Al Galaa Street
Cairo

The Middle East Observer
41, Sherif Street
Cairo

EL SALVADOR
Fusades
Alam Dr. Manuel Enrique Araujo #3530
Edificio SISA, ler. Piso
San Salvador 011

FINLAND
Akateeminen Kirjakauppa
P.O. Box 128
SF-00101 Helsinki 10

FRANCE
World Bank Publications
66, avenue d'Iéna
75116 Paris

GERMANY
UNO-Verlag
Poppelsdorfer Allee 55
D-5300 Bonn 1

GUATEMALA
Librerias Piedra Santa
5a. Calle 7-55
Zona 1
Guatemala City

HONG KONG, MACAO
Asia 2000 Ltd.
46-48 Wyndham Street
Winning Centre
2nd Floor
Central Hong Kong

INDIA
Allied Publishers Private Ltd.
751 Mount Road
Madras - 600 002

   Branch offices:
   15 J.N. Heredia Marg
   Ballard Estate
   Bombay - 400 038

   13/14 Asaf Ali Road
   New Delhi - 110 002

   17 Chittaranjan Avenue
   Calcutta - 700 072

   Jayadeva Hostel Building
   5th Main Road Gandhinagar
   Bangalore - 560 009

   3-5-1129 Kachiguda Cross Road
   Hyderabad - 500 027

   Prarthana Flats, 2nd Floor
   Near Thakore Baug, Navrangpura
   Ahmedabad - 380 009

   Patiala House
   16-A Ashok Marg
   Lucknow - 226 001

   Central Bazaar Road
   60 Bajaj Nagar
   Nagpur 440010

INDONESIA
Pt. Indira Limited
Jl. Sam Ratulangi 37
P.O. Box 181
Jakarta Pusat

ISRAEL
Yozmot Literature Ltd.
P.O. Box 56055
Tel Aviv 61560
Israel

ITALY
Licosa Commissionaria Sansoni SPA
Via Duca Di Calabria, 1/1
Casella Postale 552
50125 Firenze

JAPAN
Eastern Book Service
Hongo 3-Chome, Bunkyo-ku 113
Tokyo

KENYA
Africa Book Service (E.A.) Ltd.
Quaran House, Mfangano Street
P.O. Box 45245
Nairobi

KOREA, REPUBLIC OF
Pan Korea Book Corporation
P.O. Box 101, Kwangwhamun
Seoul

MALAYSIA
University of Malaya Cooperative
    Bookshop, Limited
P.O. Box 1127, Jalan Pantai Baru
59700 Kuala Lumpur

MEXICO
INFOTEC
Apartado Postal 22-860
14060 Tlalpan, Mexico D.F.

NETHERLANDS
De Lindeboom/InOr-Publikaties
P.O. Box 202
7480 AE Haaksbergen

NEW ZEALAND
EBSCO NZ Ltd.
Private Mail Bag 99914
New Market
Auckland

NIGERIA
University Press Limited
Three Crowns Building Jericho
Private Mail Bag 5095
Ibadan

NORWAY
Narvesen Information Center
Book Department
P.O. Box 6125 Etterstad
N-0602 Oslo 6

PAKISTAN
Mirza Book Agency
65, Shahrah-e-Quaid-e-Azam
P.O. Box No. 729
Lahore 54000

PERU
Editorial Desarrollo SA
Apartado 3824
Lima 1

PHILIPPINES
International Book Center
Fifth Floor, Filipinas Life Building
Ayala Avenue, Makati
Metro Manila

POLAND
ORPAN
Palac Kultury i Nauki
00-901 Warzawa

PORTUGAL
Livraria Portugal
Rua Do Carmo 70-74
1200 Lisbon

SAUDI ARABIA, QATAR
Jarir Book Store
P.O. Box 3196
Riyadh 11471

**SINGAPORE, TAIWAN,
MYANMAR,BRUNEI**
Information Publications
    Private, Ltd.
02-06 1st Fl., Pei-Fu Industrial
    Bldg.
24 New Industrial Road
Singapore 1953

SOUTH AFRICA, BOTSWANA
For single titles:
Oxford University Press
    Southern Africa
P.O. Box 1141
Cape Town 8000

For subscription orders:
International Subscription Service
P.O. Box 41095
Craighall
Johannesburg 2024

SPAIN
Mundi-Prensa Libros, S.A.
Castello 37
28001 Madrid

Librería Internacional AEDOS
Consell de Cent, 391
08009 Barcelona

SRI LANKA AND THE MALDIVES
Lake House Bookshop
P.O. Box 244
100, Sir Chittampalam A.
    Gardiner Mawatha
Colombo 2

SWEDEN
For single titles:
Fritzes Fackboksforetaget
Regeringsgatan 12, Box 16356
S-103 27 Stockholm

For subscription orders:
Wennergren-Williams AB
Box 30004
S-104 25 Stockholm

SWITZERLAND
For single titles:
Librairie Payot
1, rue de Bourg
CH 1002 Lausanne

For subscription orders:
Librairie Payot
Service des Abonnements
Case postale 3312
CH 1002 Lausanne

TANZANIA
Oxford University Press
P.O. Box 5299
Maktaba Road
Dar es Salaam

THAILAND
Central Department Store
306 Silom Road
Bangkok

**TRINIDAD & TOBAGO, ANTIGUA
BARBUDA, BARBADOS,
DOMINICA, GRENADA, GUYANA,
JAMAICA, MONTSERRAT, ST.
KITTS & NEVIS, ST. LUCIA,
ST. VINCENT & GRENADINES**
Systematics Studies Unit
#9 Watts Street
Curepe
Trinidad, West Indies

UNITED KINGDOM
Microinfo Ltd.
P.O. Box 3
Alton, Hampshire GU34 2PG
England

VENEZUELA
Libreria del Este
Aptdo. 60.337
Caracas 1060-A